Dr

MW00893735

The Ultimate Dream Interpretation

Guide

Uncover the Hidden Meanings of

your Dreams

Written By

Mia Rose

Mia Rose

Contents

Introduction

I want to thank you and congratulate you for getting the book, *"Dream Interpretation for Beginners – Uncover the Hidden Meanings of Your Dreams"*.

This book contains proven steps and strategies on how to interpret the meanings of your dreams.

Using traditional dream meanings passed down through the centuries, this book will teach you the basics of dream interpretation. The book looks at how the meaning of dreams has been a subject that has fascinated all human cultures, including our own. It examines why we place such importance on our dreams and what they may be able to reveal to us. The book explores which dreams may have important meanings and those that don't. It also looks at the key meanings that occur in many dreams relating to love, money and career. Along with the traditional meanings described here, the book also looks at how those meanings can be interpreted in the 21st century.

Thanks again for reading this book, I hope you enjoy it!

Chapter 1: Dreams; A Very Human Mystery

The meanings and understanding the meanings of dreams has been a preoccupation of humanity since, as far at it is possible to tell, we really first became human. While some supernatural or "occult" areas of study have been firmly dismissed by modern science, the study of dreams is one area in which science, or more specifically psychoanalysis, has continued to show much interest.

The human brain and the mind retain a level of mystery, even for scientists, and while techniques such as MRI scanning have allowed for a greater understanding of the physical makeup of the brain the true nature of the mind still remains, to a large extent, still shrouded in mystery. Psychoanalysis itself is a young science with beginnings only in the last hundred or so years. Humans, and their dreams, have however been around for much longer.

Today, many psychologists believe that dreams play a significant role in the workings of our mind and in contributing to our mental and emotional health. They seem, as far as can be established to help our brain to process the day's events, perhaps help us to work out difficult problems (both emotionally and practically) and appear to have a function for transferring knowledge and information into our unconscious or subconscious mind.

The latter function makes sense; our short term memory can only store so much information but much of what we learn in life needs to be stored "somewhere". It seems that our brains use a number of process to place important information, possibly everything we experience into the archive that is our unconscious mind. It's also understood by many psychoanalysts that this information affects our behavior even when we don't "remember" consciously the information stored in our brain.

Throughout our lives, as we store more information, our brain begins to build and notice patterns in life and in events around us. This may explain the way in which we instinctively understand what will happen next in many situations; our brains appear to forewarn us with complex and sometimes confusing dreams of coming events. In this context there is little that is occult or otherworldly about interpreting dreams and it can be seen as an expression of the sheer power of the human mind.

However modern science and psychology view dreams, historically, they have been viewed as significant. In the past they have often been variously seen as signs and omens. In many cultures they were (and are) viewed as direct messages from the dead, or from divine beings. People who experienced vivid dreams were considered especially blessed and, in many civilizations, those who could "interpret" dreams were seen as holy or revered individuals.

Interestingly, in both ancient traditions and modern science, although the theories differ, nearly every culture in both the past and present has given significance to dream meanings. They may expose our inner selves, our fears and desires or they may give us valuable information and insights which seem almost to have an occult source. Either way, few people do not attach meaning in some sense to our dreams.

So how much, or which version of our understanding of dreams is true? Perhaps none or perhaps something of many different theories has truth in it. Dreams are not unique to humans and many animals also appear to regularly dream. Dreams certainly seem to have some function and as science is only just beginning to truly explore the incredible power of that marvelous organ the "brain" perhaps, in time, a better understanding of how dreams function and what they truly are will become apparent.

One thing is, however, clear; dreams are extremely visual in their nature. They can be short snippets of images or feel like feature-length movies. They are rarely in print form and often not only (or purely) verbal. Dreams are about images and there may well be a good reason for this. Humans are intrinsically visual and sight has been one of the most important senses to us for much of our evolution. Our brains are wired to receive visual information far better than any other type of information.

Every other form of communication, more or less, we need to learn but (for most people) we don't need to learn to see. Nor do we need to really learn the meaning of some very basic symbols. We see simple things like safety and danger in color (red for danger, blue/green for safety). These symbols are almost universal. The human mind needs visual signals and stimuli to remember, interpret and understand. This may explain why our dreams are so very visual and often, very symbolic. They employ archetypes to get the message across to us – even if we don't want to hear that message!

Can Dreams Tell the Future?

Yes, no, maybe; dreams do, at times, seem to be able to do this. Some people may have more vivid and apparently psychic dreams than others. However, in some sense, dreams can be said to make, or influence, the future. A very strong dream, just before you wake, will leave a strong impression on your mind. It may seem strange, unlikely and the events may seem random (that, unfortunately is how dreams work!). However, in the following day, or days, events may unfold that bring the dream back to us. It will almost certainly (and however resistant to the dream you are) work on some level to govern your responses to those dreams. Whether this is an example of psychic ability or, more likely, an example of our brains working in a powerful way to bring about the results that we desire, we have yet to fully establish.

Whatever your view, dreams have for much of human history been used to understand ourselves better and to help us to see or foresee what is coming in life. This book takes a look at the common symbols found in dreams and the meanings that have been attributed to them over many hundreds of years.

Dream Interpretation; The Rules

The first rule of dream interpretation is to trust yourself! The second is to think before you interpret! The definitions in this book are taken from a wide variety of sources and many of them have been passed down from different sources, books or traditions over many centuries. Our dreams are very personal to us and the symbols that appear may mean something deeply personal to us, or may represent cultural archetypes. Interpreting dreams can take a little time and thought – what do the symbols and events in the dream relate to in your own life? When using the meanings in this book, try to place them in context within your own life.

As an example, imagine a dream in which you see a black-smith smash your smart-phone to pieces! Centuries ago a blacksmith would be a common sight and a smart-phone would have been witchcraft (some might still view them that way!). Today, the opposites (more or less) apply!

You could look at the "meanings" for these symbols in this book or choose to interpret the meanings in relation to yourself. In centuries past a blacksmith was considered magical – perhaps a folk memory from very ancient times where these mysterious people turned stone into iron. That cultural mystery and sense of "otherness" remains and has found its way into more than one movie. However, real black-smiths are rare creatures today and if you dream about one think about the wider meaning described in this book. In this dream the meaning could be that magical, external forces, creative forces, or even authority figures, are interfering with your ability to communicate! However, always interpret in the context of your own life; if you *are* a blacksmith, or know one, be more careful where you put your phone in future!

In short, always look at what the symbols in your dream mean to you. The meanings in this book relate to archetypal images and their most likely cultural meaning for many of us.

Dreams that Matter and Those that Don't

Traditional dream interpreters ascribe different levels of importance to different types of dream. They define three main categories and these are;

- Physical dreams; these are inspired by your physical health. If you are ill, your dreams may become confused or even delirious. In this category other physical stimuli can be included such as eating too much before bedtime! Usually these dreams occur early in the night and can be largely ignored.

- Dreams of memory; these are simply memories from the past that you relive in your dreams and they can be fairly obvious to identify. They may have no significance or they may represent issues that you need to deal with. Consider the dream, the impact it has on you, and the issues it's exploring.

- Dreams of significance; dreams *after* midnight are said to have more significance than those before. In our early stages of sleep we are "processing" the day. Later in the night our brain is organizing and analyzing information. This seems to be the time when it recognizes patterns and is when what appear to be "predictive" dreams may occur. Our brains are putting into place all the information we have stored up and they may, at this time, find answers to problems or foresee the likely outcome of current events most clearly. Traditionally, the later a dream occurs, especially if it occurs close to waking or after our normal waking time, it is the most important dream to heed.

Some sources suggest that dreams are governed by the law of contraries; for example, dreaming of a birth means a coming death or winning the lottery means losing money. However, most ancient sources agree that this is not the case; dreams tend to mean what they say. Working out *what* that is, is the hard part!

Recurring Dreams

These often are taken to have significant meaning and, perhaps, this is a fair point. They can be good or bad but usually indicate that our brain has something it wishes us to resolve. In many traditions a dream which comes three times in a short space of time is considered to be the most significant type of recurrent dream. These dreams are also, according to both tradition and anecdote, most likely to be warning dreams. Whatever the dream, the simple rule is to take heed if it repeats several times in a short space of time.

How to Use This Book

There are certain things in life that are universal to us as humans for survival. Our ancient brains often focus on these elements in life. The signs and symbols that our brains use seem on many occasions to fall into certain categories; food for our survival, shelter from the elements or danger and relationships. Food and shelter are our basic needs, while avoiding danger and finding safety in numbers have been human survival strategies since before we were fully human. Dreams that relate to these elements of our lives are significant, perhaps the most significant. In this book we use these basic categories and explore the most common meanings found throughout history, relating to them.

Chapter 2: Dream Meanings; Food and Sustenance

Sustenance is important to us all and dreams sometimes use obscure symbols to get their meaning across when relating to this subject. A dream about eating a delicious meal with a loved one may relate more to the meaning that we have a fulfilling relationship than to what is on the plate. Lack of food, or someone taking food from your plate, may not be about having a bad experience at a restaurant but simply suggest that the relationship with the person in their dream is not giving you what you need! Always be aware that dreams will use symbolic people. Eating with a parent (alive or dead) may symbolize authority or it may symbolize support and protection from the parent in question – or that you still have such support in life. In this section we'll look at some common, accepted meanings related to consuming food and drink.

Alcohol, Drunkenness

Though this may be related to real life events, beer, brewing or distilling were symbolic of many different things in many cultures. In many, brewed or distilled drinks were safer than water to drink and this cultural element may linger in some people's folk memory. Generally, brewing is a sign of success, but after delay. Drunkenness is variously interpreted as loss through foolishness or confusion and delays brought about by your own actions. Much depends on the context of this dream but it is generally a warning.

Banquets and Feasts

Food, in a party context in general, is to found in this category of dreams. If the celebrations go well and the food is plentiful this is a sign of success, often in work and business as well as in context of good friendships. If you see others eating but are not doing so yourself this is a sign of success to come but after a delay. Lack of food and/or a bad atmosphere indicates coming disappointment and possible failure. Generally, plenty in any sense in life is indicated by feast where large quantities of good food are available but the opposite is indicated where food is scarce or poor quality.

Bottles and Drinking Vessels

Generally, this is a sign of plenty and good fortune. If the liquid in the container is clear, pleasant and palatable, this means general good luck and indicates you have resources which will bring you strength. Broken drinking vessels indicate loss and poverty and may indicated broken or lost promises. This can relate to personal relationships, your own security or to work situations.

Butter

Commonly considered a positive omen, your efforts have been rewarded and completion, success and fulfillment are indicated by this dream. Modern day alternatives are included here! Any food which smells bad, is distasteful or dangerous indicates a negative outcome and in this case it suggests you fear that your efforts have been wasted.

Cakes and Confectionery

Considered, almost universally, a positive omen, especially for the young and for those embarking on new relationships. Plenty, comfort and happiness are all symbolized by cakes and confectionery.

Cheeses

Considered negative in dreams by many older sources, suggesting disappointment or loss. Some believe this may indicate a need to make detailed plans and be prepared for a long wait to see the results of your effort.

Cereal Crops

A very ancient and significant symbol, corn-fields, wheat-fields or other fields growing crops of any kind, are considered to be very significant dreams. They symbolize, when healthy, plenty, riches, wealth, good investments and even status. The stage of growth indicates where you may be in this cycle. Failed crops and diseased plants suggest the opposite but may act as a warning to look at your plans. Crops, today, can include houseplants, or parks and gardens, as fewer of us are involved directly with agriculture!

Eggs

Once a staple food and a valuable replaceable source of protein. Eggs also symbolize birth, beginnings and potential in our minds. Eating eggs suggests you have created solid foundations for growth, buying or selling them suggests profit and good fortune. Broken eggs foretells bad decisions and loss. Much, in this case, will depend on the specifics of the dream and other symbols within it.

Fruit and Nuts

These are symbolic of good fortune, plenty and rest and relaxation in life. Like all foods the meaning can depend on the quality and quantity of the food. Bad, or lacking foods, mean lack of positive feelings in the area they relate to.

Meals

Different meanings have often been ascribed to different meals throughout the day. Breakfasts, especially plentiful ones, suggest energy and, in particular, mental energy; they indicate beginnings and the stamina to take initiative with these. Lunch suggests plenty in many traditional sources (breakfast and an evening meal were more common for most people in history). Evening meals suggest positive conclusions and an successful completion of projects. Again, much depends on the quality and quantity of the food and the company you keep in these dreams when interpreting them. Dreams about mealtimes are negative if food is bad, limited or arguments break out.

Milk

As with eggs this was, and is, an important commodity in many cultures. Meanings are very similar for both eggs and milk, success if you are drinking milk is usually indicated. Material gain and good fortune are generally associated with milk. Where the milk is bad, many sources suggest bad fortune. Some suggest that this may indicate you should look to use the resources you have in new, innovative ways.

Ovens

Including just about all manner of cooking implements. Generally this type of dream is considered fortunate. A hot oven with food cooking suggests plenty, good fortune, comfort and stability. It also suggests projects brought to fruition. Cold ovens, or empty pans suggest lack of resources in some area of life but are most often considered to suggest opportunity, new starts and that chances are coming that will allow you to create success. Negative aspects of this symbol include broken ovens or other cooking equipment, or ones that will not cook, despite apparently working. This suggests projects (or relationships) which you are trying to manage in the wrong way, with the wrong tools.

Chapter 3: Dream Meanings; Jobs and Money

Jobs and money, to most of us in the modern world, are primarily linked to our security and this in turn relates to the very basic human need for shelter. Whether you have a job to pay the bills or a career that you love, either way the issue of your security and ultimately shelter are strongly implicated in this area. In this section we'll take a look at some of the most significant dream interpretations relating to this need.

Ball Games

Many dream interpretations connect games, and ball games in particular, with financial affairs and employment. If you dream of having a ball thrown to you and catching it, this suggests coming opportunity and success. Be prepared! If you fail to catch the ball, or it rolls away from you, the meaning is generally interpreted as still being fortunate but you will face delays and missed opportunities before success is achieved.

Banks or Banking Transactions

If another person receives money through a bank or through a banking transaction in your dream this is a sign of disappointment, delay and failure in your endeavors. It may suggest that you are not being recognized, in some area of life but usually a work related area, for your efforts. Work here can mean employment, business or charity. To receive money in a dream is generally considered a good omen. It suggests promotion, new projects which will be successful and recognition for your hard work.

Beacons

A beacon, or any bright, shining, directional light, including lighthouses and or the headlights on vehicles is a dream of good fortune and prosperity. It often suggests safety, security and the end and completion of projects in a successful way. Bright lights generally signify safety and security but also an indication that you will receive help from others to bring about that result. It's also considered a strong indication of passing troubles and hope for the future. The dream may indicate that although prospects seem bleak, inspiration is at hand to turn a situation around.

Bees

Symbolically bees are signs of hard work and achievement. Success is nearly always indicated if you dream of bees; in most cases this will be through sheer determination, attention to detail and hard work. A small number of bees indicate these are the qualities you must learn to apply now while a larger number suggests your efforts are close to reward and you have the skills you need already. To be stung by a bee or bees indicates almost exactly what it suggests, the hard won success may come at a cost in other areas of life and may be barbed with regret.

Counting

Linked to success and accumulation, but if you make mistakes during the process this suggests a delay before both are achieved. A warning to be scrupulous and pay attention to details is often suggested in this case. Business projects will soon show positive results if the counting is easy and accurate. If it is slow and labored, much work will be required to achieve your goals.

Communications

Letters, emails, texts, phones, the Internet and social networks can all be included in this category! Dreams about communication were, at one time much simpler – usually referring to letters or telegrams. However, the basic rules apply in whatever form you dream about communication! To see somebody else reading a letter meant for you (reading your texts, hacking your Facebook account!) warns of betrayal in some form or other. This usually indicates the breaking of promises or secrets being exposed. Dreams connected to communication generally relate to emotions

Mia Rose

and relationships but can also relate to business. In this context, seeing another read your "letter" may suggest you are giving too much away, or have rivals seeking to better you by deceit. Receiving a "letter" in most contexts means news of coming change – this can be positive or negative and may depend on the context in the dream.

Fabric

Any kind of fabric is often related to business and work related ventures. Good quality, beautiful or intricate fabrics indicate positive outcomes, success and abundance. Poor quality suggests there is some flaw in your endeavor. New fabrics suggest opportunities will come to you soon and you would be wise to take them. Old fabric suggest that whatever you are working on has had its day – it's time to move on.

Royalty

For the modern world we should include political leaders here as well. This is generally considered to be both a sign of great fortune close at hand and general prosperity. It's also considered to suggest a rise in status (promotion is a strong possibility). This dream warns of coming opportunity and it usually does refer to the world of work and business; the opportunity may seem too good to be true when it comes but this dream advises you to take it.

Towers

Including towering buildings of all kind. Symbols of strength, power and defense, dreams in which you enter and climb a tower suggest projects that will come to success. Much will depend on the nature of the dream and your relation to the building. If you encounter difficulties in climbing the building this suggests success is possible but you must take care in your approach. Broken, or falling towers, are signs of sudden change of fortune (usually but not always) in a negative way. Towers under construction (especially if you're involved) denote hard work but great achievement is promised.

Treasure

Digging for treasure (or winning the lottery) is a complicated dream – and a very old one. It has a number of meanings and much depends on the context. It can mean fruitless labor – and in a business sense this can mean you should consider your next move or the usefulness of your current role/project. If you find treasure this usually indicates that your labors will be rewarded in the end – but the search or the effort could be long. Generally considered a warning that there are easier ways to achieve the goal for which you are aiming.

Volcanoes and Earthquakes

Another strange dream which can relate to any area of life. In terms of work and business this is a sign, not surprisingly, of sudden change. Dormant volcanoes indicate danger and trouble ahead, which may overtake you suddenly (redundancies, closures, lost orders or legal problems). Active volcanoes and earthquakes suggest that the time for action (probably change) is now. The dream usually relates to events which are beyond our control. This dream is a warning, in most cases, to be prepared! The dream itself is not necessarily a bad dream but indicates that you sense something is "wrong" with a situation. The outcome can depend on your response in the real world.

Chapter 4: Dream Meanings; Love and Relationships

Humans are social animals, perhaps the *most* social, and our survival has long depended on our ability to build relationships with other people. Whether that's in the context of work, play or at home our relationships with others define us. Most of us are deeply intuitive (whether we realize it or not) when it comes to our personal relationships in every area of our life. We know when something is "wrong", when something is "right". This is instinctive and it comes from years (tens of thousands of them) of experience. Our intuitive knowledge is often buried deep inside our unconscious minds – how often have you felt uncomfortable around a new acquaintance or associate for no "reason"? On most occasions your first instinct will have proved right. In our dreams, signs and symbols will frequently appear that will "tell" us things we need to know about our relationships. They can be both positive and negative and usually it's wise to take note of them. In this chapter we'll look at some of the ways in which our brain most commonly tries to get these messages across.

Altar

Generally, to dream of a wedding is a sign of disappointment. Contrary though this may seem, most sources agree on this. This can be interpreted as misplaced trust or of promises that may not be kept. In other contexts an altar symbolizes judgment in some form and indicates that you should search your heart for your true feelings – generally in relation to an emotional situation.

Beauty

In any form, this is a sign of love and happiness. If you are beautiful yourself in the dream it suggests a happy love life and one with great potential. To see beautiful people in your dream is a sign that you are loved very deeply. It is also considered to be a sign of great success in area of life but is particularly related to relationships – be they with partners or friends.

Candles

A very, very old symbol which we can substitute for "light sources" in all their modern variety. A bright candle, or light, tells us that we have a trustworthy friend or companion who is watching over us. A low, faltering light (guttering candle in older sources) suggests that gossip and rumor is being spread about you. Friends may not be what they seem in this case.

Crowds

Generally, a good dream which foretells good times around the corner, parties, holidays, friends and happy friendships. The nature and mood of the crowd should be taken into account but generally this dream suggests good times, social events and happiness. This can even be true if the crowd seems hostile; in this instance you may be feeling nervous about an event but the dream suggests that your fears are unfounded.

Father (or Father-figure)

Whether your real father is alive or dead, dreaming of an individual who fulfills this role for you is considered to be a very significant dream indeed. If the father offers advice it should be heeded, if he seems happy or sad try to understand the source of this emotion. Whatever this figure expresses take note as it's likely to be an important message that your brain is trying to get across to you. Dreams of this nature can be very personal to the individual and deserve attention and thought as to their true meaning.

Jewelry

To dream of wearing jewelry indicates that you have an admirer who has yet to make them-self known to you. This is considered a fortunate dream in many respects and the brighter or newer the jewelry appears the more likely that you will discover who your admirer is in the near future.

Tarnished, dirty or damaged jewelry is still believed to denote an admirer but the individual may be less than trustworthy. This dream may be a warning.

Mother (or Mother Figure)

Much the same as father, this dream is also seen as a promise of help and loving friends. If you are facing problems or worries you will find help readily given. This may come from your real mother or it may come through close friends or relatives. This dream suggests that you should confide your worries in someone you trust and help and solutions will be found. As with a father-figure dream this can be a very personal dream but nearly always suggest selfless support is available should you choose to seek it.

Moonlight and the Moon

Dreaming of the moon is considered to be a sign of great good fortune for those in love. If the moonlight is clouded it is still considered a good sign; though troubles may loom in the future, they will pass. In general this is a sign of great good fortune in love and of happy outcomes in romantic relationships.

Music

To dream of music is believed to suggest that you will hear from old friends or reconnect with people who are important to you. Its a sign of friendship but especially of the renewal of friendship. If the music is sad this can be a sign of problems with a friend and the possible loss of that friendship. It's often a dream of significance, whichever the case, and should be acted upon quickly.

Religious Figures

To dream of any religious figure is, in many traditions, taken to be a sign of coming disappointment in a relationship. Be careful of the context here; if you are planning to be married the dream is less likely to have any significance other than you will, in many cases, have to deal with a figure of this sort. If you aren't planning (or already are married) the warning of disappointment is likely to be more significant.

Water

Water is an element strongly associated with emotions; water in this sense can mean ponds, pools, baths, rivers, streams or whole oceans. To dream of clear calm water suggests all is well in your relationships. To dream of dark, stormy or muddy water suggests trouble in your personal life. Traveling over stormy water indicates the most difficult problems. Unclear water suggests that there are secrets or hidden elements to the trouble. The outcome of the dream is often important, stormy waters becoming calm means a

Mia Rose

positive outcome is on its way while the opposite means there is trouble brewing.

Chapter 5: General Dream Symbolism

Dreams are all about symbols; as stated earlier in the book we are very visual creatures. This is our intrinsic and default nature; we can communicate with anybody from anywhere by using symbols, images and signs. In the twentieth century, when man first began to explore beyond the planet on which we live, spacecraft set to travel beyond our own solar system were sent off containing images on the basis that intelligent life elsewhere in the universe would understand symbols rather than be easily able to decipher our languages.

In this final chapter we'll explore common symbols in the context of our dreams. These images may have very specific meanings in your own life but many are universal to all of us. One area where some "messages" from the brain may not be universal is the symbolism behind colors. The meaning and association of some colors is different in different cultures; in many western cultures, for example, red is associated with danger, but in China and other eastern cultures the color is associated with good luck and prosperity. This book focuses on dream interpretations in the western tradition – if you're cultural background is none-western, consider the implications of colors in your own culture when interpreting your dreams.

Colors In Dreams

In this section we'll look only at the black, white and the primary colors red, blue and green. Other colors are a combination of these and the influences of each color will be "colored" according to their predominance. Many people don't dream in color and when colors dominate a dream it is often an important sign, which suggests the dream is of strong significance.

- Black; traditionally associated with bad news, loss or grief, black can also mean change and secrecy. Major changes in life (hence the association with death) are often signified if a dream is "colored" by this tone. Death itself is not necessarily indicated but can be interpreted as the death of ideas, or a relationship. Generally, the color warns that big changes are either coming or are needed in your life.

- White; as with black this is a color that has been associated with mourning (in both western and eastern cultures). In traditional interpretations the color is seen to indicate change, in much the same way as black. It is also seen to indicate a "blank canvas" and represent opportunities to begin a new chapter in life. The color also symbolizes purity, newness, beginnings and honesty. However, some sources state that where white dominates a dream it can indicate a "white-wash" - that things are being covered up or that secrets are being kept. Interpreting this kind of dream can be complex and white has associations with spirituality; it can suggest the hidden, the unknown and new opportunity all at the same time. Often the best advice to take from this dream is that you have the opportunity to begin afresh but should take care to establish facts.

- Black and White; generally this is taken to suggest that you are seeing things in real life in black and white! This can be a warning that you need to view a situation with more objectivity and awareness that there are possibly many different perspectives on an issue or situation. Consider the message of the dream carefully and look for alternative views or advice on the matter that the dream seems to be related to.

- Blue; this color suggest wisdom, honesty, intellect, peace and creativity. This is the color of clarity of thought and can suggest that you need to bring your intellectual capabilities to the matter at the heart of the dream. Blue has another side to it – the color of the oceans and water it relates to deep emotional contacts and bonds in a positive way. Blue indicates that you have good friends or loved ones in your life and indicates peace and happiness in matters of the heart.

It indicates honesty and trust in personal relationships.

- Red; traditionally this is interpreted as a warning in
  dreams. Red indicates danger, anger, destructive
  tendencies and sudden change. It has associations
  with fire – which can be both destructive and renew-
  ing. Some sources ascribe passion and energy to red
  as a color and it can certainly indicate this in dreams.
  Many dreams featuring this color call for swift, deci-
  sive and clear action over the matter in hand. Darker
  reds suggest anger, particularly suppressed anger,
  while lighter tones, those towards oranges and pink
  foretell the potential for powerful, rapid changes.
  Very vibrant reds can warn that you may need to stop
  and think about your actions before taking them.

- Green; the associations of green for most of humanity
  are positive. The color indicates fertility, growth,
  prosperity and abundance. This can be in any or all
  areas of life. It can signify a coming birth, a change
  (for the better) in circumstances. Darker greens suggest things coming to fruition, to completion and the
  reaping of rewards after labor. Lighter greens suggest the beginnings of new projects that will be successful. Growth, fulfillment and personal achievement are all signified by this color and it many cul-

tures it is strongly associated with good luck. Darker shades of green have also long been associated with financial prosperity.

Death in Dreams

Death is a fundamental fear in humanity and it appears in dreams in many guises. However, it is not, traditionally, believed to interpret impending death either of the dreamer or the person dreamed of. To dream you see yourself dead, often indicates a sudden change of circumstances (this can be positive or negative) and a leap into the unknown. If you see another person dead this can indicate impending illness, or betrayal in a friendship or relationship – the individual may become "dead" to you. Generally, dreams in which death appears to feature are a warning of some kind that change is on its way or is urgently needed. To dream of death is not, however, a negative dream at all, it simply strongly suggests change and this change can often be for the good.

Landscapes

Landscapes appear in all of our dreams. They can be familiar places or places that we know that take on different, unrecognized forms. Sometimes we dream of specific landscape features; woodlands, mountains, open countryside and cityscapes. The meaning of the dream is often impacted by the nature of the landscape, if it feels threatening it is a warning, while a pleasant landscape indicates positive outcomes. The following symbolic landscapes often appear in dreams, although the meanings should be, again, interpreted in some context with your own life.

- Forests and Woodlands; forests were the wild-lands, filled with fear, danger and uncertainty for our ancestors. They were places to avoid, places of mystery and confusion. In a forest it is impossible to get a clear sight-line, and between the trees, it can be hard to make out what that movement from the corner of our eyes was. However, forests were also strongly associated with the "other" in this sense meaning other worlds, the spiritual and the divine. In our dreams forests and woodlands can have both of these meanings. Generally, if the forests or woodlands in our dreams are dark, tangled and intimidating places this suggests fear, anxiety and a sense of lack of control. They are strongly indicative that we feel lost, cut off from society, or alienated in some sense. Searching for a loved one in a forest indicates you feel cut-off from them, have lost a sense of connection or simply lost contact with them. Being hunted or chased in a forest can mean you have enemies in some area of your life; or that others are deceiving you, leading you down false paths or leading you astray. Bright, sunny, lush forests have very much the opposite meanings to the former. Usually this type of dream features more open woodland. This dream has associations with peace, with a deep spirituality and connection to your inner self. If you feel confident in the setting this is a sign that you will prosper in life and that you will draw on your own inner strength, belief and creativity to achieve your ends. This is a very positive dream for artists, scientists and also for new parents! This is a dream that indicates independence and self-reliance and tells us that we have enough of both to make a great success of our lives.

- Mountains; a mountain or mountain range has a number of different meanings in dream interpretation. In many cultures mountains were, like forests, wild places and often were obstacles to travel. In dreams they can be placed in several contexts. If you are climbing a mountain this means that you must make great effort to achieve your goals, the road is likely to be long and dangerous. Much will depend on your own emotions and attitude in the dream. To struggle and give up means that you are unwilling to preserver in your task – and it may not be worth it. To continue on doggedly can indicate you have the strength and stamina you need. To reach the top of a mountain suggests success – great success – but this may depend on the view. If it's clear, wide and spectacular you will – after effort – achieve your dreams and goals in life. Obscured or cloudy views, in this case, mean that the efforts you are making will not bring positive results or that they will not be worth the effort you have invested. Dreams relating to mountains can relate to any area of life – relationships, finances or career. They indicate great obstacles which must be conquered and the outcome of the dream can offer you insight into whether or not you should pursue the course of action you are currently on.

- Open Countryside; again, common in dreams, but with very variable meanings. The underlying message in this dream is opportunity and particularly the opportunity for success. As with mountains, this can relate to any area of our life. Career and wealth are often associated with dreams of open landscapes but all areas of life can be indicated. Much will depend what is currently on your mind or the focus of your life. The appearance of the landscape and the conditions of both the weather and your own attitude are the key points to take note of if this type of dream occurs. If you feel threatened, exposed or afraid of the landscape this can indicate that you are holding yourself back in some way – that opportunity is there but you need the skills to take it and, importantly, the courage to do so. Where you feel confident and safe within the setting the dream indicates that you have the skills to make the most of the opportunities that come to you. This dream is extremely lucky and promises success in many areas of life. Where the landscape appears overgrown, neglected or the weather conditions make it threatening, this is a sign that much work is needed to bring your opportunities to fruition. It can also indicate that you are not making the most of your skills, talents and the opportunities that present themselves in life. Take this dream as a warning – you have everything you need for great success but are not using it to your best advantage. Open countryside of fields filled with ripening or ripened crops is also an excellent omen, success in this case is very close at hand.

• Cities and Cityscapes; cities are very new additions to the landscape in terms of both the planet's history and human history. They are indicative of order, civilization of wealth, opportunity and relaxation and ease in life. They are also highly symbolic of commerce and trade. While dreams in cityscapes often indicate business, work and wealth they can also relate to other areas of life. Today, most of us live in cities or urban environments and the meaning of dreams relating to them may also indicate our homes, security and safety.   Generally, as with many dreams, our attitude and feelings towards the city in the dream indicate the meaning of the dream. Where we feel happy, comfortable, safe and familiar with a city, this suggests real opportunity and prosperity in matters relating to work, business, trade and new ventures. It is also suggestive of good friends, of so-cializing of opportunities to enjoy ourselves. Cities can be strongly representative of our civilized side. If you are happily exploring a strange city consider this a sign that new interests and valuable opportunities are coming your way. When negative, a cityscape will look dangerous, rundown or a feeling of being lost or fearful will dominate the dream. This indicates that we are concerned about our jobs, our careers or that we have deep rooted fears of interactions with others. We may have taken business decisions (or be about to) that we have misgivings about. We may lack much connection in our lives with culture or civiliza-tion and need to connect more with the outside world.

Conclusion

Thank you again for reading this book!

I hope this book has given you insight into your own sign of the Zodiac and that of your friends and family and also highlighted some areas which are overlooked in modern Astrology.

Finally, if you enjoyed this book, please take the time to share your thoughts and post a review on Amazon. It'd be greatly appreciated!

Thank you and good luck!

Preview of Chakras For Beginners

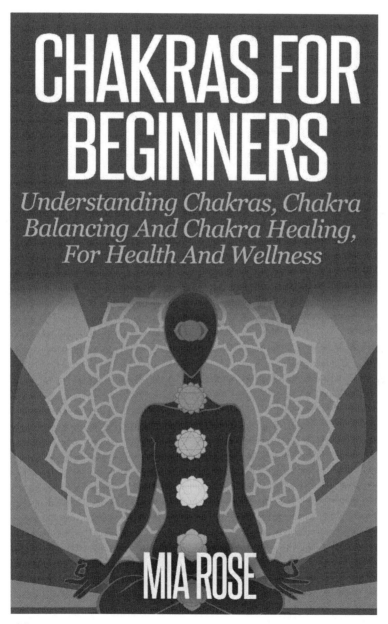

The ancient study of Chakras has made its way into the western world as of late. Frequently the first exposure can come through the study of yoga, meditation or Hindu practices.

The body and every living being is filled with a universal energy that connects and surrounds us. This energy can has been described as being made up of 7 layers (Auras) and the 7 chakras (energy points or knots in the body)

This book is designed to offer a practical, usable introduction to the Chakras, how they can affect our health and well-being and how to identify imbalances and address these.

The book is designed for those new to the concept but will also be useful for those with some experience of Chakra and energy healing. In the next chapter we take a more detailed look at what the Chakras are, and an overview of each one of the seven main Chakras. The remaining part of the book looks at each individual Chakra and how to examine the Chakra for imbalances. The final chapter provides a simple list-style section of tools that traditional (and modern) Chakra experts believe are useful in achieving balance within your Chakra energy system.

When our Chakras are in balance they allow energy to freely flow through our bodies and keep us revitalized, healthy and connected to the world around us. However, imbalances within the Chakra system can cause the energy to become blocked, leading to ill health both physical and emotional.

Here Is a Preview of What you'll Learn...

- History Of Chakras
- What Chakras Are
- In-depth Description Of Each Chakra
- Causes Of Chakra Imbalances
- Chakra Test
- How To Balance Each Chakra

Click here to check out the rest of Chakras for Beginners on Amazon.

Check Out My Other Books

Below you'll find some of my other popular books on Amazon and Kindle. Check them out by clicking on the images. Alternatively, you can visit my author page on Amazon here.

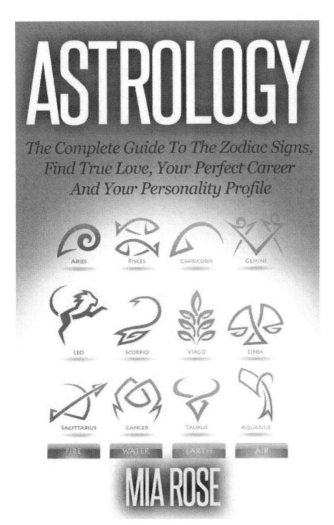

http://www.amazon.com/Astrology-Complete-Perfect-Personality-Horoscope-ebook/dp/B00N6HWV6K

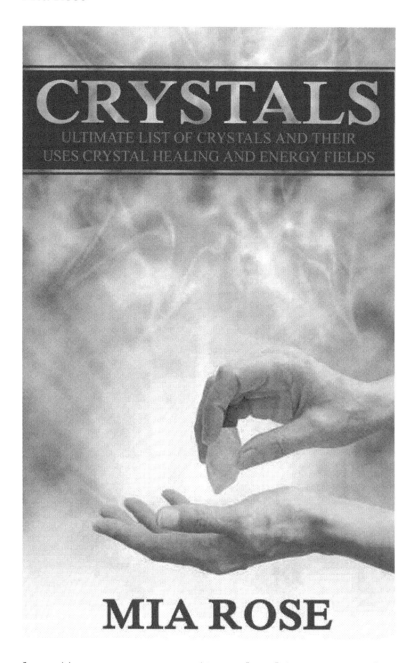

http://www.amazon.com/Crystals-Ultimate-Crystal-Healing-Spirituality-ebook/dp/B00SWMDP46

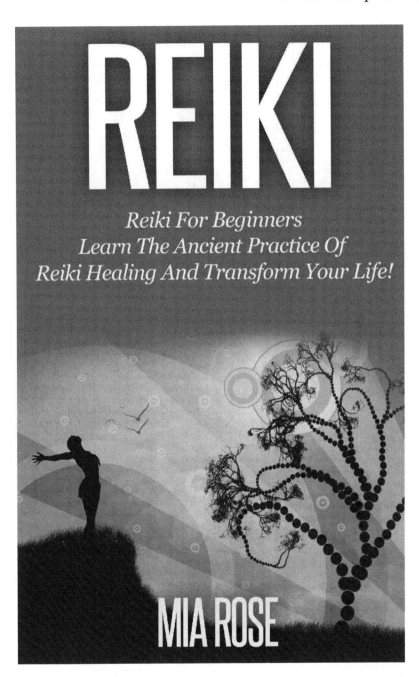

https://www.amazon.com/dp/1502391678

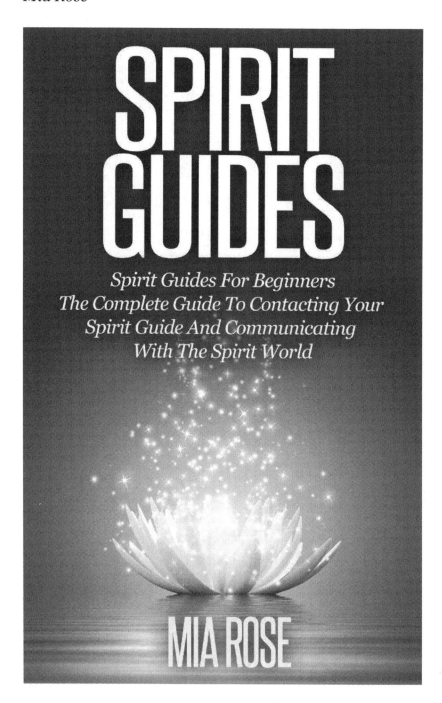

https://www.amazon.com/dp/1502502186

About the Author

I want to thank you for giving me the opportunity to spend some time with you!

For the last 10 years of my life I have studied, practiced and shared my love of spirituality and internal development. I kept diaries for years documenting the incredible changes that graced my life. This passion for writing has blossomed into a new chapter in my life where publishing books has become a full time career.

I feel extremely blessed and fortunate to have the opportunity to share my message with you! Each of my books are written to inspire others to explore the many aspects of their internal world. My goal is to touch the lives of others in a positive way and hopefully be the catalyst of positive change in this world :)

Mia Rose

I am forever grateful for your support and I know you will get immense value through my books. I am really looking forward to serve you and give you great insight into my passions!

Your Friend

Mia Rose

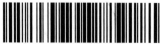

21637184R00031